Notes / Ex

FROM THE

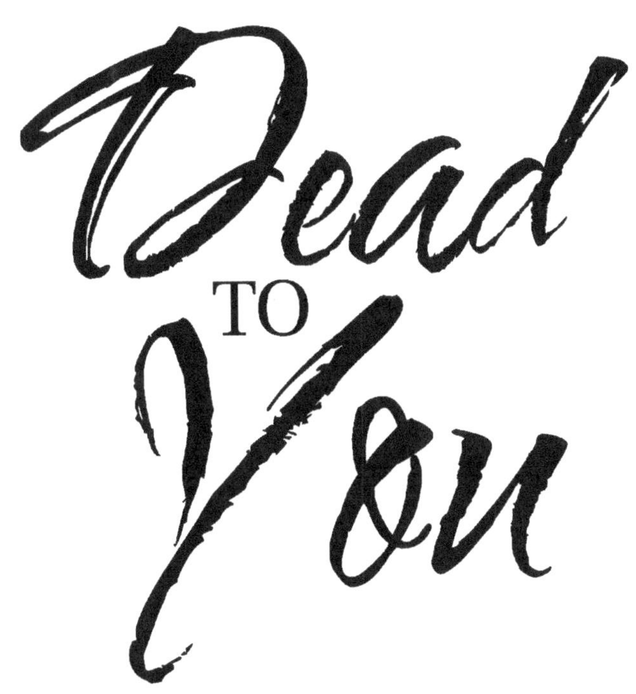

Dead to You

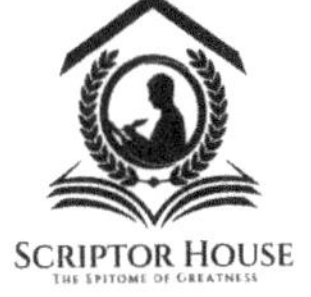

SCRIPTOR HOUSE
THE EPITOME OF GREATNESS

CAROL LEE

Scriptor House LLC

2810 N Church St Wilmington, Delaware, 19802

www.scriptorhouse.com

Phone: +1302-205-2043

Published by Scriptor House LLC

Paperback ISBN: 979-8-88692-188-5

eBook ISBN: 979-8-88692-189-2

Introduction

It's been many years and many days,over a thousand bodies later, when I have finally realized that there are many things to laugh about in life. In death. I am being asked almost on a daily basis: how did you get into this line of work? My answer has always been: I did an elective and spent two weeks in the morgue, and I knew that I could do this for the next 20 or so years. The truth is that I stumbled into it. Just like you stumble into anything in life, really. Many of us spend hours watching television shows/documentaries about crime scene investigations and autopsies, but how many are given the opportunity to stumble into the real thing in life? For that, I am thankful. It has made me realize that big things in life cannot be planned, just lived. Planning really just involves the little things such as when and where to have dinner, when and where to bring my children to skating lessons, and so on so forth. Death (suicides aside), is one of those big things that cannot be planned. It just happens.

I always wonder what people's last thoughts were just before they died, and whether or not they knew at that moment, that moments later they were going to die. Would you be thinking about family and friends, things that could be done when you had the chance to, or just about yourself?

With that, I start to write. About people, who are no longer with us. One at a time, day after day, month after month.

Wedding bells

34-year-old male and 32-year-old female. Cause(s) of death: Multiple blunt force injuries.

What's more romantic than getting engaged and moving on, having a vision of the future and some concrete plans? A nice dinner at a nice restaurant, a man proposing to a woman, the woman being the love of his life. The woman said "yes", and off they went walking into the sunset. Little did they know, as they were strolling leisurely down the sidewalk, that a swerving vehicle driven by a drunken driver would appear behind them and sweep them off their feet (and into the air/ground/whatever was around) to eternal bliss? Just like that.

It happened quickly (which was good news).And both of them succumbed to death (which was also good news). They could be any of us. The drunken driver could also be any of us. Maybe they are now planning their wedding or living their future in a better place. And who knows, the drunken driver may have learnt his lesson, received his penance,and gone on to become someone useful in life. Mistakes are made, people die. If this is a story that can make you re-think what you want to do or not do in life, just remember, there is no guarantee when or where your life will end.

Personal demographics are altered to protect case confidentiality

Mr. & Mrs. Smith

Can you love someone so much that the feeling of not being loved in return turns to hate? A young married couple resided in a moderately furnished home, with pictures of them happily together plastered on every inch of their walls. It was a usual evening, when the wife dutifully prepared dinner for the two of them. They sat opposite to each other, enjoying their food quietly, contemplating on their respective events of the day. The husband finished his share, got up, and obtained a second serving. The wife, also having finished her share, sat quietly across from him, watching him eat. She started making comments about him neglecting to obtain a second serving for her. And hence began a verbal fight. Verbal fight turned into physical altercation, and at some point, she took a knife in her hand and stabbed. One stab was all it took, and he collapsed.

Clearly, the triggering event is trivial, although it is the top block of a tall stack of blocks, which happens to be the one that tips over the entire tower. A problem only becomes a problem if you let it grow. Maybe some things are better addressed when they are small, so that your blocks do not get piled too high too fast for your tower to crumble. If you feel like you are crumbling inside with the most trivial of encounters, maybe it is time to dissect and deal with your issues one at a time, five minutes at a time. And talk about it. Out loud. With someone you trust and love. Before love turns to anger or hate.

** Personal demographics are altered to protect case confidentiality.**

Family values

22-year-old female. Cause of death: Drowning

Tis the age to fall in love. Tis also the era of free love. At least that is what most people believe. A young girl fell deeply in love with a person of a different ethnic background, whom her family strongly disapproved. And so the story went: argument after argument, lie after lie, evasion after evasion, secret after secret, and one day, something snapped. She took a walk along the riverbank, contemplating why the world had to portray love one way, and why her family viewed love as something entirely different from how she felt it. She could not understand why something as pure as two people falling in love could receive such a lack of blessing from people who claimed to love her and to want the best for her. She thought that he was the best that had ever happened to her. In her family's mind, she had done something so terribly wrong that could not be forgiven, and with time, she began to believe it herself. That it was unsalvageable. Love was unsalvageable. And she walked further and further, and further, and further, into the water. It felt cold. But not as cold as she felt.

Having family values is a good thing, and it is something that we should pass on to our children. However, when things do not go as planned, do we have a plan B in mind? Do we have an open mind at all? Or do we blindly pursue these so-called values? What this family did not know at the time was that they were not losing a child, but also an unborn grandchild. Maybe she was over-reacting, but "all is fair in art and love". Did she love him enough to warrant these actions? Only she herself and God would know.

**Personal demographics are altered to protect case confidentiality. **

Saving face

It was New Year's Day when he was found face down on the floor by his spouse. Or at least that was what she claimed. Standard procedures followed, with investigators questioning members of the family to get more information surrounding the circumstances and his medical history. Nothing of note came out and he was believed to have succumbed to natural causes, except for one detail. His neck was surrounded by a deep-set line that was unexplained. More questions followed, including those concerning symptoms of depression or suicidal thoughts. His spouse firmly denied, claiming that he would not bring shame to the family this way. More authoritative bodies were notified, including the police, which eventually brought the family to the police quarters for formal interrogation. Only then, the family confessed that he indeed had been exhibiting symptoms of depression, and that he was in fact found with a string around his neck.

Is depression shameful? Is sickness or death itself shameful? Would you deny someone close to you treatment for a potentially treatable condition for fear of exposing their condition to others? Some things are better left unsaid, but some things may get better when brought to light. Let's hope we all have the wisdom to differentiate between the two.

New Year's Day signifies new beginnings. And maybe, just maybe, for him and for his family, this was a new beginning.

**Personal demographics are altered to protect case confidentiality. **

Why me?

A new life, a new start, a new hope for everyone. In some cultures, sleeping with tummy-side down is advocated (some babies even like this position) so that the baby's soft skull will not take on a flattened back. It was an ordinary day, when his mother had breastfed him and put him down for a nap, tummy-side down. He normally slept tummy-side up at night, and tummy-side down otherwise. It had been 4 months and he had been feeding and growing well. Everyone was happy, except for the fact that he was found unresponsive about an hour later when his mother checked on him. A complete autopsy, review of circumstances, and review of medical history did not reveal a pertinent cause of death, and he was deemed to have died of what is currently known as sudden unexpected infant death (a condition that is multifactorial, meaning with no one concrete causal factor but rather involve multiple factors at play, and is associated with various risk factors that are observed in a number of anecdotal cases). Risk factors for this condition include sleeping tummy-side down (or prone).

Why me? But he had been well before, why now? The answer is, nobody knows. And like many other things, knowledge as it has developed up till this day has failed to explain many phenomenons. We, as humans, attempt to explain things all too often to cope with life's ups and downs, but how many of those explanations can be truly proven right or wrong? Life goes on no matter what, and if you find yourself ruminating over something that ultimately you won't know the true answer to, maybe it is time to move on.

**Personal demographics are altered to protect case confidentiality. **

Forgive and forget

88-year-old female. Cause of death: Blunt force
head injuries

It was just another day for her, residing in her care facility which cared for elderly residents, many of whom had dementia, a condition that affects memory, language, and cognitive functions for daily living. A fellow friend and elderly resident came up to her and pretended to play a game of football with her, and body tackled her. She fell, in turn hitting her head, causing significant internal bleeding. She was alive and well one minute, and unresponsive the next.

Who is to blame? The demented resident who thought he was just playing (and likely had already forgotten the event shortly after)? The care facility for not watching their residents diligently and following them around at all times? Or the decedent for appearing at the wrong time in the wrong place next to the wrong person? Dementia is a cruel disease, robbing you slowly of not only your memories, but also your dignity. However, there is a lesson to learn in every experience, and this time, it may well be to forget and forgive.

**Personal demographics are altered to protect case confidentiality. **

Halloween fright

22-year-old male. Cause of death: Gunshot
wound of head

It was the one day of the year when you could have blood on your face and not be out of place. He had picked this one day for effect. He had never messed anything up. He had been a straight-A student, and had spent all his life making his parents proud. He attended a most respected university. He joined the most respected teams and societies. He made sure that he appeared composed and happy at all times. There were times when he thought he could not do this anymore, but he pushed on, always challenging himself for higher achievement, and not to disappoint. Even till the last day. He knew he had to do this perfectly. It had to work. He thought that he'd better do some planning and research on his part.

Bullets came in boxes, but all he needed was one, if he did this right. He left the receipts of his purchases (gun and bullets) on the bed, and loaded an instruction manual on "how to use a gun" onto his computer screen. It was his first time using a gun, and his last. One shot, just as he wanted. Another success to add to his list of achievements.

It is shocking how some people can push on for a long period of time without showing any overt signs of dysfunction, all the while accumulating so much negative energy within that they accept the negative energy as part of their lives. Suicidal thoughts are no longer impulsive. They become part of their grand plans. It is one thing to end a life on impulse, but it is something entirely different when thought and effort are being put to work, in aims to end a life -- it becomes a first degree murder, to oneself. If you are in such a situation, please stop yourself from committing murder, even if it is just to oneself.

** Personal demographics are altered to protect case confidentiality. **

New Year's Resolution

20-year-old male. Cause of death: Mixed drug toxicity

It's that time of the year again...a time to reflect, correct, and resolve issues in preparation to start a new page. As a young vibrant 20-year-old, he thought he could take over the world. There were thousands of opportunities and possibilities, and it was the age for experimentation to find oneself. It was New Year's Eve afterall. Loud music, dancing, and alcohol were more of the norm than the exception. And despite regulations, some partiers always managed to smuggle various prescription and non-prescription drugs into the party grounds. Taking one pill made him high, taking two pills made him higher, taking three just about made him forget who he was. Maybe that was what he wanted. He did not want to know what was in the pills, just as long as they exerted their advertised medicinal effects, and all his friends were taking them. He danced lighter, expressed himself a bit easier, and thought that he was more of who he wanted to be. So why not take more? Before long, he started feeling dizzy, had a bit of a headache, so he decided to find a quiet corner to sleep it off. His snoring was drowned out by the loud music and noise around him. He had no recollection of when the party ended, for he never woke up.

It is nice to be young. I remember those days. You are eager to throw yourself out there thinking that you are invincible and undestroyable. Some survive, some don't. But let's never forget that you are human afterall, and what you do to your body is going to affect you and the people around you. There are other ways to be cool. Drugs is just not one of them.

** Personal demographics are altered to protect case confidentiality.**

More New Beginnings

It's New Year's Day, let's talk about life instead. I was once called to the labor and delivery suite to deliver a 10-pound baby from a 21-year-old mother. It was her first baby and first babies usually take longer to deliver. So there I was, semi-coaching her through her labor, and all I could think of was how amazing this young lady was. She was completely focused on the process, followed instructions extremely well, and did not make a sound! She had a slim frame so her belly looked disproportionately big on her.

Somewhere during this process, the father of the baby walked in. Big muscles, long graying hair, clad in a biker vest, arms covered with various tattooed motifs. He also had a persistent frown on his face. I am human afterall and made a silent judgment: how did this beautiful young petite lady end up with this aging gruffy-looking dude?

And then something miraculous happened: the baby came out, and the mother breathed a sigh of relief. It was the father who sobbed with the baby in his arms, while he kissed the mother tenderly, with all the emotions you could have wished for in a father. The mother was calm and methodically followed the staff's instructions of how to feed and care for the baby, while the father seemed to just fall head over heels over the both of them. Somewhere during the process, they would catch sight of each other and smiled. And there and then, I saw love.

Lesson learned? Never judge a book by its cover, for its contents often exceed what you expect.

**Personal demographics are altered to protect case confidentiality.*

Anger management

40-year-old female. Cause of death: Multiple blunt force injuries.

It was a nice night out for a drive. She was just minding her own business, driving along, eager to go home from a full day's work. On the other hand, in another vehicle, someone completely unrelated to her had been in a heated argument with his spouse, and got into his car in a foul mood. He decided to take it out on the street, and despite his passengers trying to get him to slow down, he swerved erratically. Why not? He was angry. He had all the reasons in the world to step on the pedal. There was nobody on this deserted street anyhow, so why stop now. He was not crazy, just angry.

And there she was, unsuspectingly emerging from an intersection, at regular speed. But he was too engrossed with his anger to notice. Nor was he able to stop at the speed that he was going. He crashed right into the mid section of her car. He survived, she died. All because of anger.

Can you imagine having to live with that kind of guilt? Actually, is it worth it to have to live with that kind of guilt? What would you do after an event like that? Those are the questions on my mind when a case like this comes by. But then again, we cannot predict what will happen the next moment, and there was a real possibility that he could have survived his momentarily irrational act with nobody getting hurt. God knows how many momentarily irrational acts we have got through in our lifetimes. The one thing we can learn from this unfortunate incident though, is that there are safer ways to let out our anger, which do not involve someone else dying.

** Personal demographics are altered to protect case confidentiality.*

Being born dead?

Imagine being sick with a stomach flu, feeling nauseated and unwell, thinking you have to go to the bathroom and all the whilenot knowing that you are about to give birth to a baby into the toilet bowl. This was the story of a 19-year-old mother, still a freshman in University, who claimed to not know that she was pregnant. No one knew what happened exactly afterwards, for she was all alone, but a friend came to her aid soon enough, which was when the baby was found in the toilet bowl, with an abundant amount of blood at the scene. No cause of death was found. There were no significant injuries, natural diseases, or toxic substances to explain his death.

Such are the challenging cases. The birthing process is complex, and can be traumatic at times to cause subtle physical or biochemical derangements thatare detrimental but not necessarily overtly visible. And then there are those conditions which sometimes do not show overt postmortem findings: did he drown, did he get too cold and become hypothermic, or did he suffer from some form of asphyxia (lack of oxygen due to airway disturbance) shortly before birth, during birth, or after birth? Short of an accurate account of the sequence of events (not often available partly due to the emotional and traumatic nature of the process), these questions sometimes remain unanswered, and thus closure remains lacking for both the mother and the people involved. Although,in most cases, instead of dealing with the grief and trying to find closure, the young mothers (and fathers) would rather forget the whole thing and move on. The power of being young, I guess.

Young women and young men out there,you are precious, and should take care of yourselves and love yourselves more than to end up not knowing how to deal with the consequences of your actions.

** Personal demographics are altered to protect case confidentiality.*

Sad story

I had a hard time finding a title for this page but it was indeed a sad story. She was a teenager, at an age where the fun came from testing out new things, flaunting new clothes, wearing new make-up, and so on. She did not feel like she was worth it. She was 400 pounds. It was hard enough to just find clothes that fit, let alone flaunting them. According to family and friends, she was well liked, and did not express thoughts of depression or suicide; however, she had a poor body image. So yes, she could have been the most optimistic person in the world, and yes, she could have told herself that it was "okay" to be overweight, but after so many rounds of seeing your friends try on new clothes, attempt new activities, and date new guys, there was a point of breakage where there was no return. She chose the swimming pool to end her life, but it could have easily happened through any other means.

Fatnesscan be acquired, but can also be partially genetic. Thinness can be acquired, but can also be partially genetic. Society has created a certain ideal for body image, and it is important to keep in mind that only a small percentage of the population can achieve that ideal. The ideal is there to encourage healthy living, but many people take it a bit too far and eventually become unhealthy, either inbody or mind, or both. Do you have a friend in need? Can a case such as one described above be remedied in any way? I don't know. All I know is that taking one small step at a time is better than taking no action at all.

** Personal demographics are altered to protect case confidentiality.*

As a post-valentine's day thought, let's not talk about death. I received an email from a friend today outlining the following pointers to reducing stress, so that we have more time for love and care, for ourselves and for others. I think we can all use one or two of these pointers and I would like to take this opportunity to share them with you. Remember: it is not how heavy the burden is, but how long you carry it for that makes it seem heavy. May all of us put down our life's stressors once in a while and give our shoulders a rest before picking them up again. Have a good Valentine's weekend.

1. Accept the fact that some days you're the pigeon, and some days you'rethe statue!

2. Always keep your words soft and sweet, just in case you have to eat them.

3. Always read stuff that will make you look good if you die in the middle of it.

4. Drive carefully... It's not only cars that can be recalled by their Maker.

5. If you can't be kind, at least have the decency to be vague.

6. If you lend someone $20 and never see that person again, it was probably worth it.

7. It may be that your sole purpose in life is simply to serve as a warning to others.

8. Never buy a car you can't push.

9. Never put both feet in your mouth at the same time, because then you won't have a leg to stand on.

10. Nobody cares if you can't dance well. Just get up and dance.

11. Since it's the early worm that gets eaten by the bird, sleep late.

12. The second mouse gets the cheese.

13. When everything's coming your way, you're in the wrong lane.

14. Birthdays are good for you. The more you have, the longer you live.

15. Breath...deeply.

16. Some mistakes are too much fun to make only once.

17. We could learn a lot from crayons. Some are sharp, some are pretty and some are dull. Some have weird names and all are different colors, but they all have to live in the same box.

18. A truly happy person is one who can enjoy the scenery on a detour.

19. Have an awesome day and know that someone has thought about you today.

AND MOST IMPORTANTLY

20. Save the earth..... It's the only planet with chocolate!*

It's my party

20-year-old female. Cause od Death: Gamma-hydroxybutyrate Toxicity.

Having just gone through another birthday and aged another year, I began thinking of how I spent the past birthdays that I have had. I can recall some pretty crazy times but none quite like this young lady, who spent her big day with various sexual partners, male and female included, while drinking and partying. May sound familiar to some. So what's the big deal, you ask?

The big deal was that she was found unresponsive in the hallway the next morning. An investigation ensued, and according to statements, she had consumed some alcohol, but she was known to be capable of holding down much more alcohol than what she had that night. So her death remained a mystery. Healthy girl otherwise, no major injuries. Her blood tests showed some alcohol, at levels that were not generally considered lethal. Her blood was also tested for a substance known as gamma-hydroxybutyrate (GHB for short), a substance normally found in the brain in small amounts, but can also be manufactured for both medical uses or illicit uses. It can be used recreationally since it can cause disinhibition and enhanced sensuality, but is also a date rape drug that can cause significant sedation at increased amounts. It is colorless and odorless so it is very easily added to drinks, and even if consumed voluntarily, often does not leave an obviously visible trace at the scene.

So girls out there, please be aware, that this is something that is very real and happening everyday. Always keep a lookout for you and your friends while partying hard.

** Personal demographics are altered to protect case confidentiality.*

Experimenting

15-year-old male. Cause of death: Asphyxia by suffocation.

He was young and curious, at the prime age of puberty, ready to explore, experiment, and try new things. Experimenting can be trying to smoke a cigarette for the first time, trying to take a recreational drug for the first time, or trying to choke or suffocate oneself to achieve a "high"...using a low oxygen state as a means of achieving excitement and euphoria. Sounds silly, right? You may be surprised to hear that there is such a group of followers, with a big proportion of them being teens/young adults.

These can take on the forms of wrapping one's face and body tightly and ultimately decreasing the amount of oxygen in the immediate environment and/or preventing effective breathing, or constrictions of varying degrees to the neck region, often accompanied by sexually oriented motives. Hormones? Maybe. Between getting high and staying alive, the choice is quite obvious, if you ask me.

Young people out there, always be aware of the consequences before trying something new, and if your first instinct tells you that the idea is simply dangerous and silly, you should trust and listen to that instinct.

**Personal demographics are altered to protect case confidentiality.*

'Tis the season to be jolly

Christmas is fast approaching, and instead of talking about another death, I want to talk a bit about Christmas shopping. It should be realized that the spirit of Christmas has its roots stemming from religion, and I am not entirely certain at what point it became a gift-giving frenzy that many people go through year after year. Do not get me wrong: I think it is a great idea, whoever came up with it first, to give gifts to those whom you treasure and appreciate, and it is not much different from giving them a birthday gift or a gift on another special occasion as a token of appreciation. However, the politics associated with gift-giving that go unsaid creep up on me at times. Never mind questioning yourself: what should I give this person? The real question that presents itself is: what will this person likely give me (if at all), and what should I give in return to not make him/her feel under-appreciated? Gift-giving etiquette, maybe? Another specialty that I have yet to learn.

Gift-giving, just like help-giving, is an art. It requires one to know another well enough to know what will strike a pleasant chord through the gift or help given. And I am not just talking about the material cost, but the sentimental meaning of what that gift or help represents. To me, it would be ideal to be gift-giving all year round, whenever something materializes that reminds you of a particular person. And not scrambling around for "appropriate" presents just because a festival is around the corner.

When in doubt, there is always the option of a charity gift card, which promotes the spirit of gift-giving to those in real need, and hopefully is a gift that is agreed upon by most to be a respectable act of kindness.

Still painful?

40-year-old female. Cause of death: Mixed Drug Toxicity

Ouch! Nobody likes pain, especially chronic pain. But such is the case for injuries to the muscles and/or bones. The pain can come and go, can last a long time, may get better or worse, or may be helped by one medication and not the other. Unpredictable, maybe that's the right word to use. Her story is one that we hear over and over and over again. She injured her back while performing work-related duties and was treated for pain. Different medications were used and dis-used, alone and in combinations, with dose increases and with dose decreases. For months. And the pain prevailed on. What was one supposed to do? She was finally hospitalized so that she could be watched while more medications (some with quite potent side effects) were tried. One morning, she was seen sleeping peacefully, and never woke up.

Such is not an uncommon occurrence, and prompts one to rethink the risks vs benefits of modern medicine on one's health. It is often hard to know where to draw the line, since there are such wide variations as to what works on one person and does not on another. It is almost impossible to know which person will benefit from any particular pain medication. Not to mention that pain is very much a subjective "feeling". What is a 1/10 level of pain for you may mean a 7/10 level of pain for me. There comes a point when one asks: is there a better way?

** Personal demographics are altered to protect case confidentiality.*